Diabetes Now Magazine

Written And Created By Cheyene Montana Lopez

Diabetes Now Magazine Introduction

I suffer from this cold blooded disease of Diabetes Type II. I fight everyday like anyone else with this nasty silent killer. I have come along ways. But to say day to day is a challenge I face. I write this magazine as a help to others out there with Diabetes Type II. Simply I encourage each and everyone never to give up hopes. The battles goes on and on like a Merry-Go-Round. I'll call it the Merry-Go-Round to living life. Our minds are a help to encourage ones self in positive thinking modes. But truly we need support and strength, that is the foundation to it all. Sometimes we often find ourselves down so far that often we might find ourselves giving up. But we cant. Granted diet and proper foods help. In the three years I've had diabetes and yes I do my homework and constant research to try to find cures which can try to bring me back to being near as normal as possible. But I still have a long ways to go before I get there. Yet often obstacles and hurdles seem to become a barrier to get in the way. I still do not think enough is being done like me with a high diabetic reading to release what drugs that can help me in which they seem to show great strides and promise to help bring Diabetes back to normality. This has got to change. Right now I am and have been trying to get on this one medicine that has been showing such an effect. But I am unable to get it. All because of red tape that is in the way or no more clinical studies on people like me with diabetes. And I know many of you whom suffer with this need it too so it may help you or cure you as well. This has got to change on the laws. We should be allowed access to such medications which I will talk more about inside on articles in this magazine.

Hopes To One Day
Again Be Normal !!!

I seek to live normal. Everyday I struggle to get up out of bed and try to find a smile. Nobody knows how hard it is to live with Diabetes Type II till they wake up and go to the doctor to find out they now have diabetes. No one knows the milestones. One of the first symptoms I had was I was sleeping too much and got tired easily. I soon had fatigue and dry mouth. Then my vision started to get blurred and all teary eyed constantly. That was not normal for me. Almost one year ago exactly to May I found myself going down in readings. My blood sugar readings went down between 200 and 100 mg ldl and even sometimes down to even less that that. And this was up till November 2012 and yet today here in 2013 which is in February that I have now gone back to over 200 and sometimes even 300 mg ldl in blood sugar readings. And I am getting discouraged and wondering and thinking what went wrong.

Every morning it is hard to wake and I struggle. I hate so much medications. I'd like to be on less medicines. You do not know what it is to have to take Prandin at 1 tablet 3 times a day and glyburide at 1 tablet two times daily or even to take atenolol blood pressure at two tablets a day and more I could name. I just hate it. Then I get to my feet and go to preparing all I need to in which to get that good old blood sugar readings ready every morning. The first thing I do is get the alcohol and six cotton swabs for cleaning the finger tip which I'll be puncturing to get blood from. And then I have four pieces of tissue in case to which after sponging again the blood wound with the cotton swab and then place the folded piece of tissue over the blood puncture wound like a band-aide. Then I get two lanclets to use out and I place into the lancer tip and clean it real good with alcohol to sterilize. And then I get the test strips out to put into the glucometer and wait patiently an hour to take because I have to let the medications take effect before the readings and last I record them into a book. Then most of all after getting my readings I have to clean the lancer and glucometer thoroughly with an alcohol swab and put all back into a case. See simply I hate puncturing my fingers everyday know one knows how sore the fingers get everyday and the puncturing hurts too.

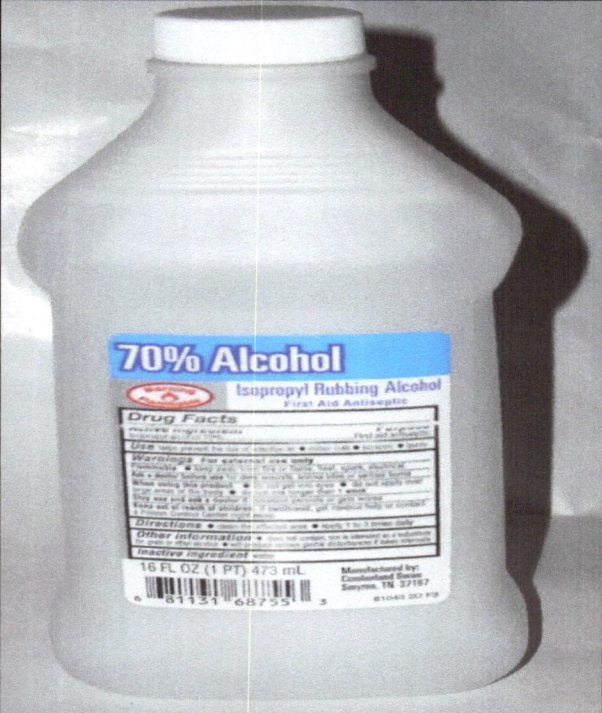

Make sure you use regular rubbing alcohol to clean with cotton swab on the fingers, tester device and and throw the bloodied swabs into a disposable container with an enclosed lid to keep down contamination.

One of the best foods my wife, Patricia A. Lopez who is also diabetic found herself are greens such as Mustard Greens, Turnip Greens, Collard Greens, Spinach, and fruits such as Un-sweetened Applesauce, Blackberries,Blueberries, Rhaspberries and vegetables are really good for diabetics. They are low in Carbohydrates and sugars. You need to find chips that have no sugar in them like Frito Lay Corn Chips, etc. Coffee is super good for you as a diabetic along with eggs, Un-sweetened teas. Search in online search engine or ask your doctors. Check the labels too for any sugar in the products.

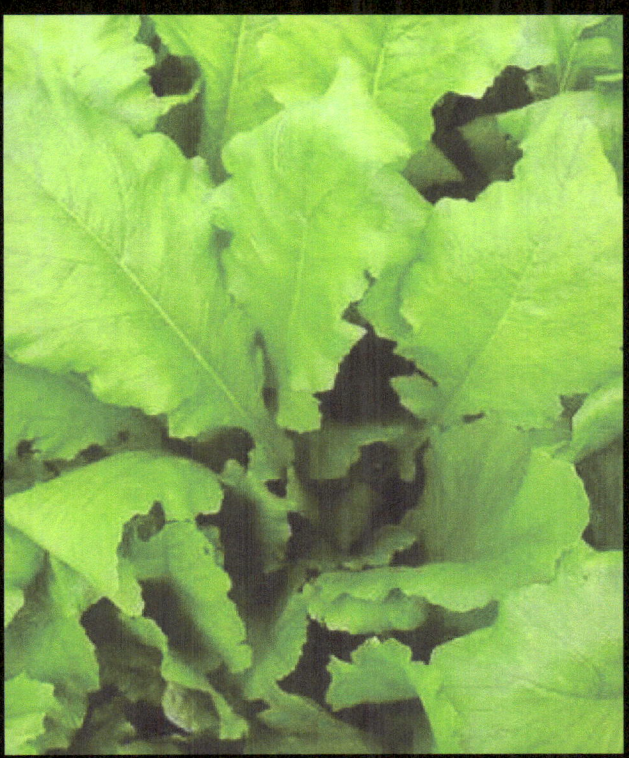

Another excellent vegetable which grows in the wild but mostly grows in the southern states is Polk Salad. You pick the green leaves and boil them three times each time in new water. Each time drain the juice off them. This removes the poison parts from Polk Salad. Once done you can find the recipe online on websites. It is very tasty to eat particularly with hot pepper juice on it. Polk salad grows on stalks and is hard to find in northern states. Sometimes grocery stores will carry the products in cans down south.

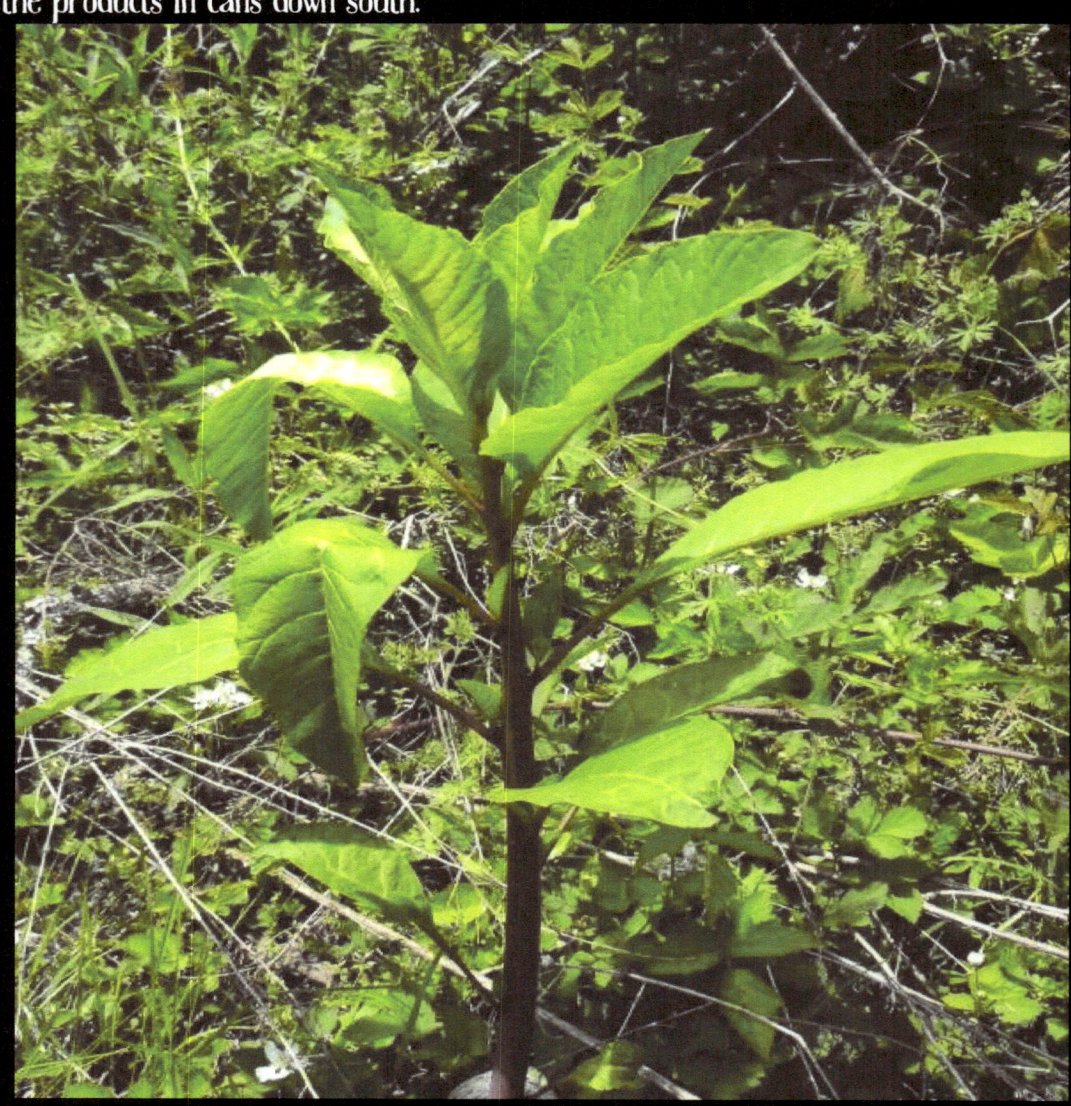

Cinnamon is an insulin substitute in Type II diabetes. Ground cinnamon helps stimulate the production of glucose-burning enzymes.In one study, volunteers ate from 1 to 6 grams of cinnamon for 40 days. One gram of ground cinnamon is about half a teaspoon. Cinnamons most impressive health benefits is its ability to improve blood glucose control. In my case of my having high diabetes readings I always take three spoons of pure ground cinnamon and trust me it really does bring my reading down. And again ask your doctors about if it is safe for you to take Cinnamon and be sure to read the labels to make sure it is pure with no sugars. Some makers do add sugar into cinnamon. Cinnamon is just one of three secrets keeping me alive.

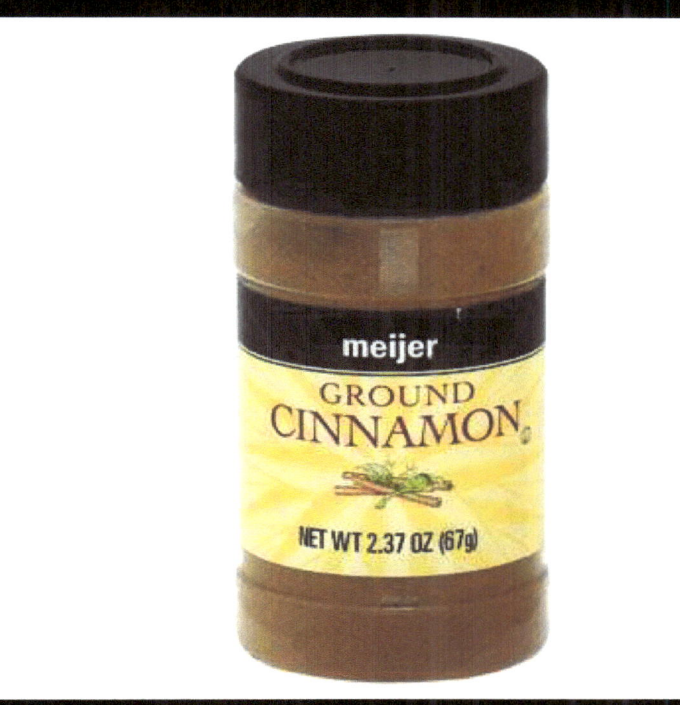

Surprise secret number two that helps is apple Cider Vinegar.In recent years, apple cider vinegar has been singled out as an especially helpful health tonic. So it's now sold in both the condiment and the health supplement aisles of your grocery store. While many of the folk medicine uses of vinegar are unproven (or were disproved), a few do have medical research backing them up. Some small studies have hinted that apple cider vinegar could help with several conditions, including diabetes and obesity. Apple cider vinegar not only is good for diabetics but also helps as a natural for acid reflux,cancer, warts, arthritis, athlete's foot, and blood pressure plus much more. Take one one small spoon full and put it into warm water or straight from a small plastic vile which you can find in dollar stores.

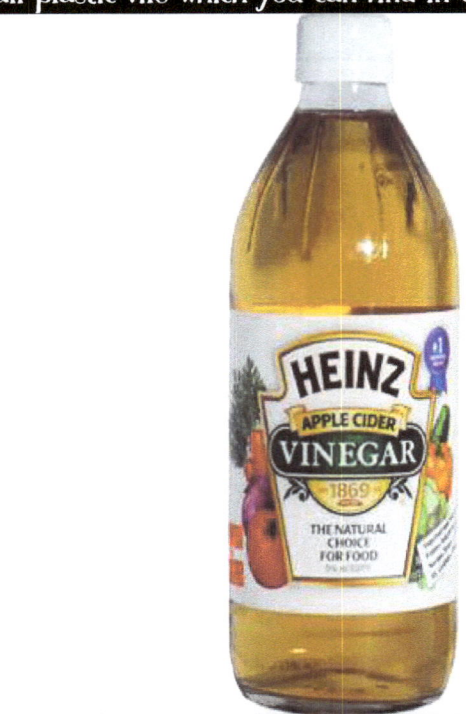

Garlic is an antioxidant that helps in treating High Blood Pressure, it helps to lower LDL cholesterol levels, reduces plaque in the arteries, Garlic helps to lower blood platelets that may cause clotting. Garlic by just taking five fresh pure cloves everyday has shown to have tremendous effects even for diabetes. Even though it can cause one to have bad breath, I'd rather have bad breath than to be dead. In my case I do not care what other people says. My life and living means more to me as well as to my wife than people. This is secret three that helps and continues to keep me alive. I also say this if you take garlic and need to be around people then you can take a half lemon and eat it or drink the juice it will remove garlic from your breath and by the way Lemons is excellent for the heart and cleaning out the arteries as well as improves breathing from the lungs.

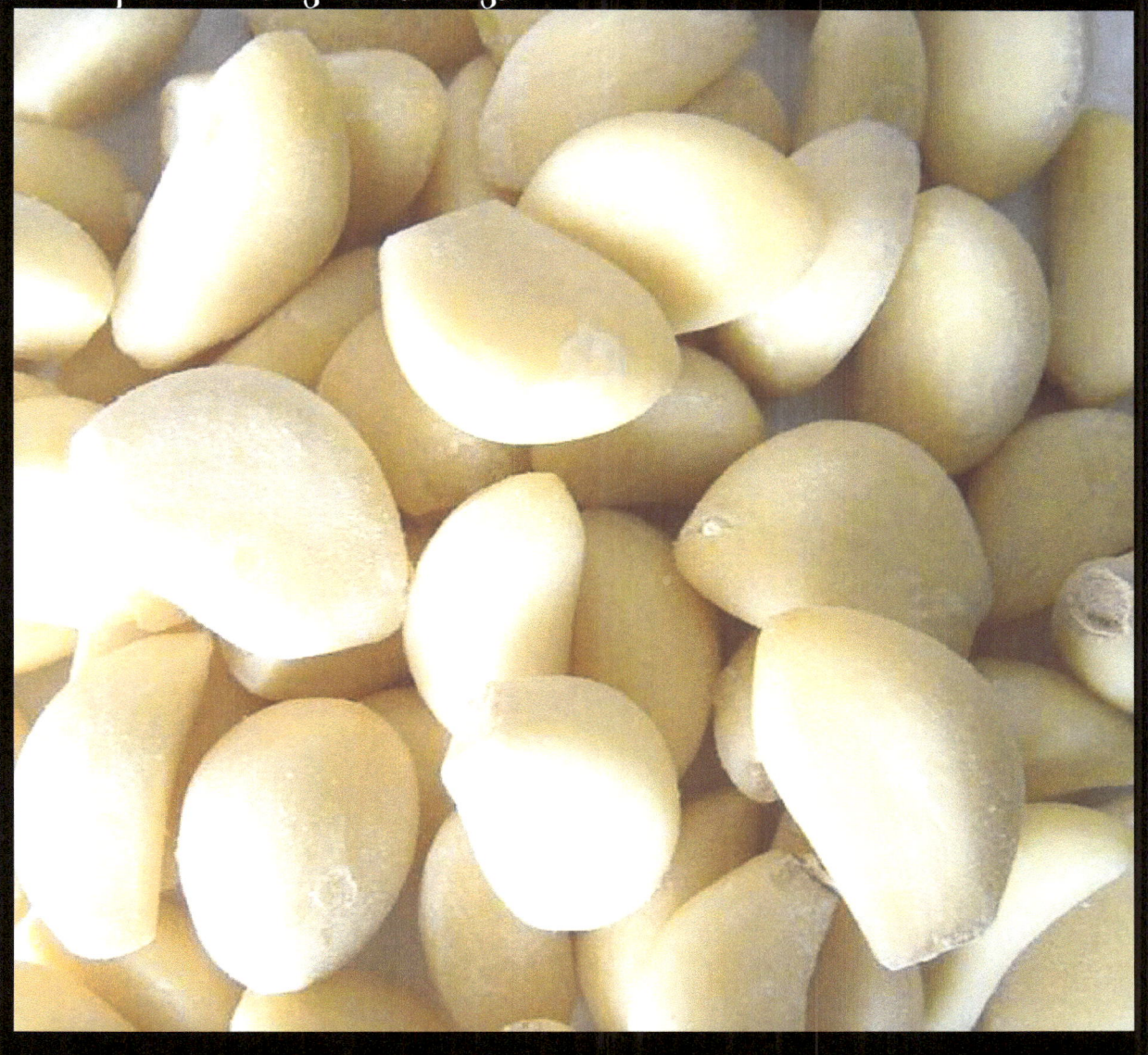

I believe keeping track of two things in life are very important and should be to everyone. 1) Blood glucometer for testing of blood sugars. 2) Digital blood pressure monitor which I believe everyone needs in their homes to check blood pressure on a daily basis. I believe laws should be changed and insurances cover this including medicaid and medicare for all including the disabled, elderly and poor. These should be given and donated for every home and are just as important as a smoke detector is. We are diabetics and we are highly as such subjects to kidney failures, heart attacks and strokes. Our goals should be to live and not put a price on a persons life. After all you could be the next diabetic or heart attack or even stroke victim.

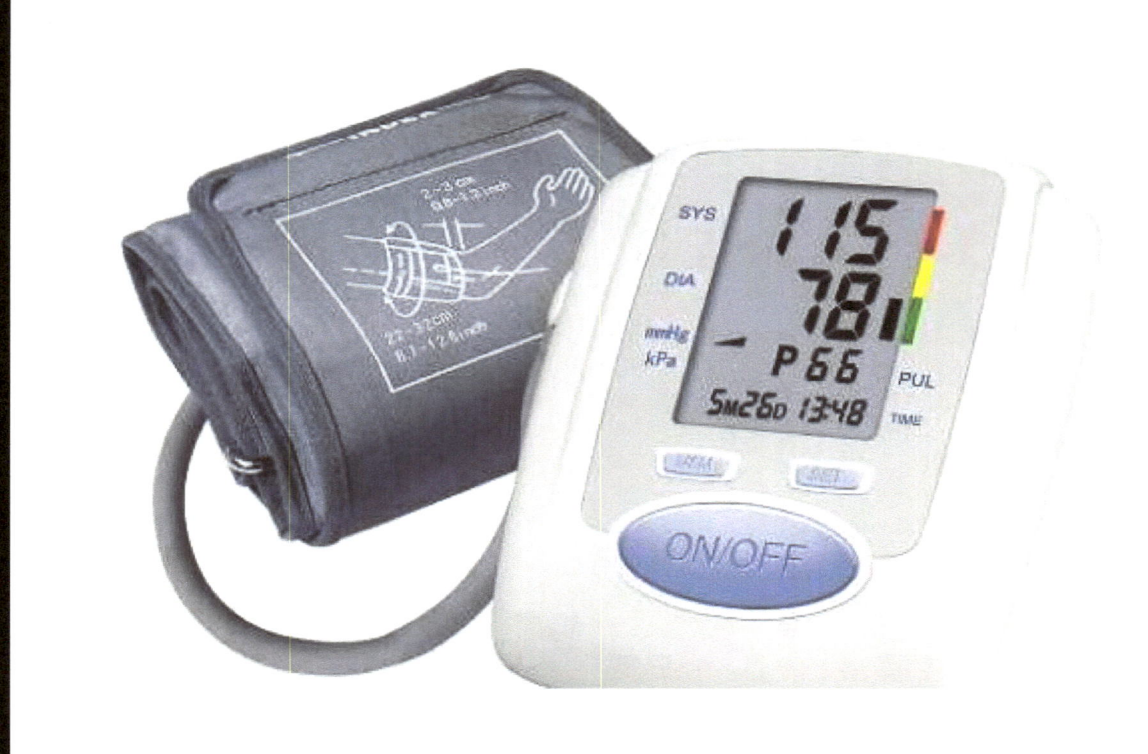

Always have a chart printed off to keep check of your daily blood sugar readings. You can find them free on most any sites online by typing in search engines such as googgle.com or yahoo.co this find free blank blood sugar charts to download for free and in case you have no printer write the website name down and link and you can go there and download and print it off for free or a little charge at your local library.

Blood Pressure Tracking Chart

Date	Time	Diastolic	Systolic	Date	Time	Diastolic	Systolic	Date	Time	Diastolic	Systolic

www.FreePrintableMedicalForms.com

Always have a blood pressure chart handy if you have any blood pressure monitor to keep records of your daily blood pressure readings for the doctor to see it. This makes it easy for you. You can find them for free to download if you have a computer and printer to print the charts off. Or in case you have no computer or printer you can again download it from the site you found and go to your nearest library to have it printed off. Be sure to have three or four printed off when printing the charts which you can find for free in online search engines free blank blood pressure charts.

DAY	DATE	BREAK FAST TIME	LEV	LUNCH TIME	LEV	DINNER TIME	LEV	BED TIME TIME	LEV

Always make sure you have lancets and plenty of test strips every months. If you are near low call the company you get the supplies from and tell them you need more test strips and lancets.

As soon as you have run out of supplies always buy at dollar stores really reasonable. You can purchase cotton swabs and rubbing alcohol for low prices. Important that you keep these on hands to wipe or sterilize with.

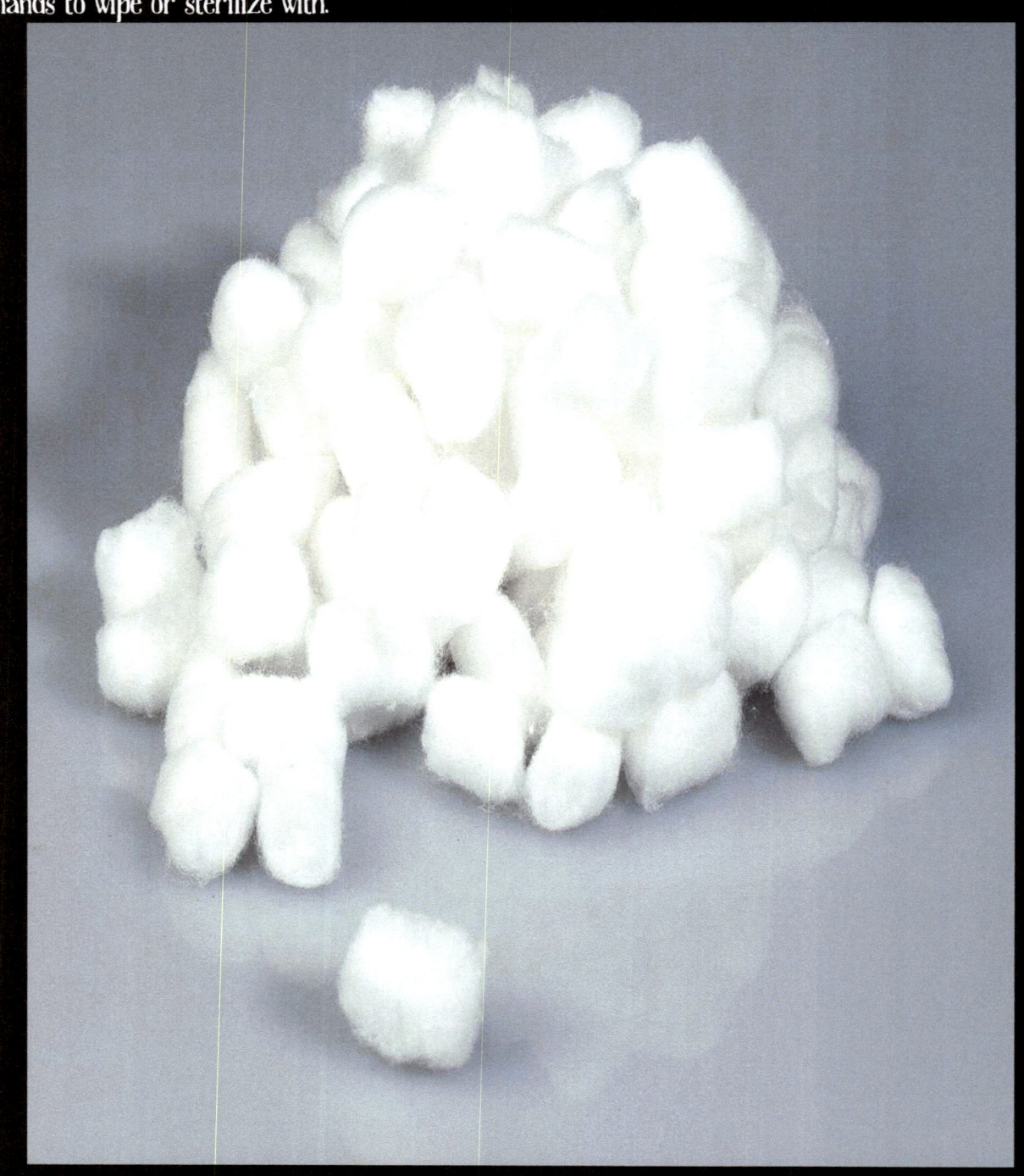

Jalapeno Peppers are enriched in vitamins. These peppers are super great for the heart among other health problems.Jalapeno Peppers contains Vitamins A,P,C & E. And if you cannot stand hot peppers to eat you can cool them down by frying them with foods like brown rice, or okra and squash fried together. However most any green peppers are good for health and diabetes too and thus pretty much contain these same vitamins.

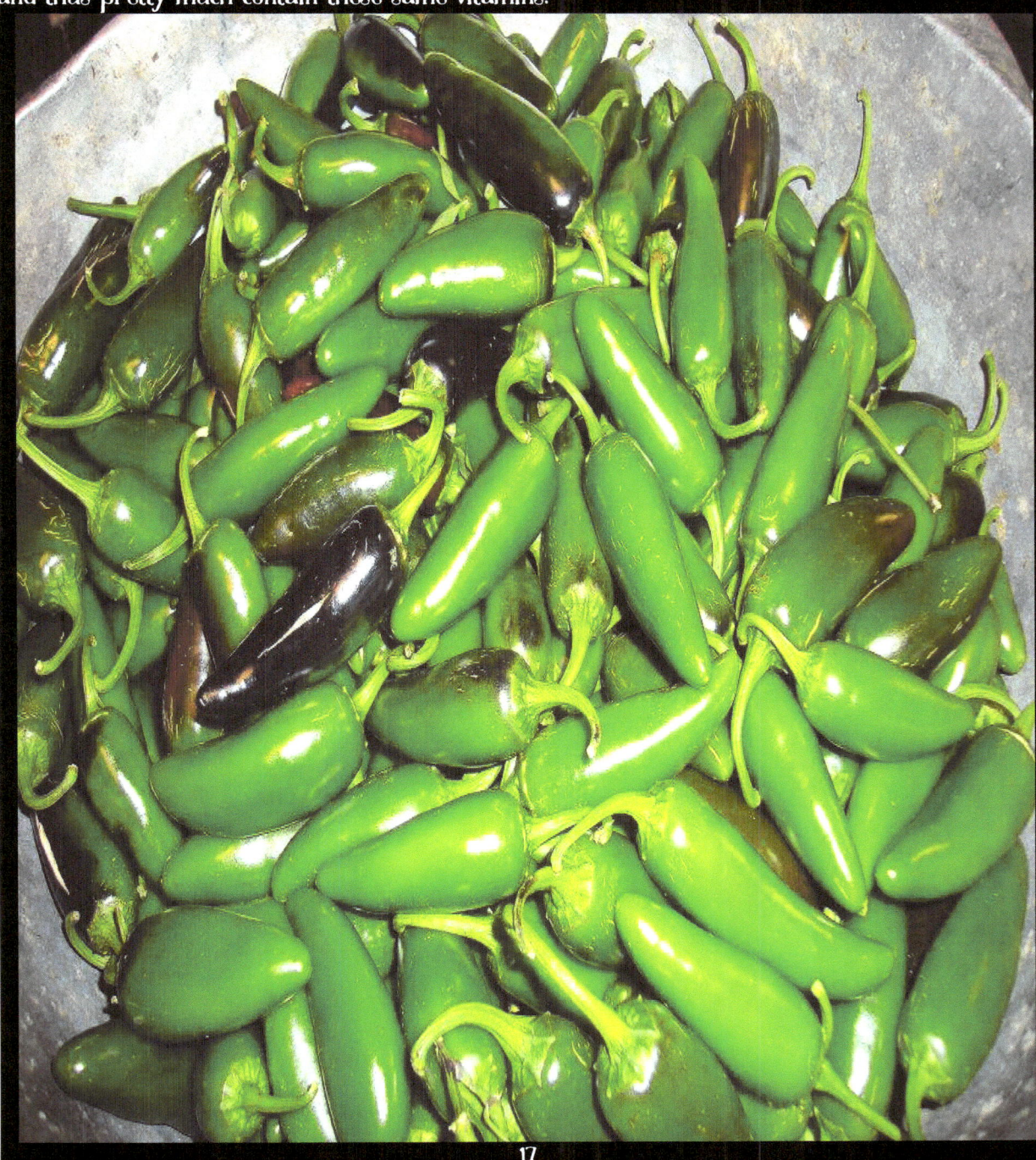

Always go to the doctors. Make sure your health is doing great and especially if you have diabetes so you can be monitored. This is so very important to do. The more you see your doctor the less likely you'll have diabetes and even this includes other diseases too. Early detection makes good health. Monitoring diabetes and having the proper medications means living and winning the battles.

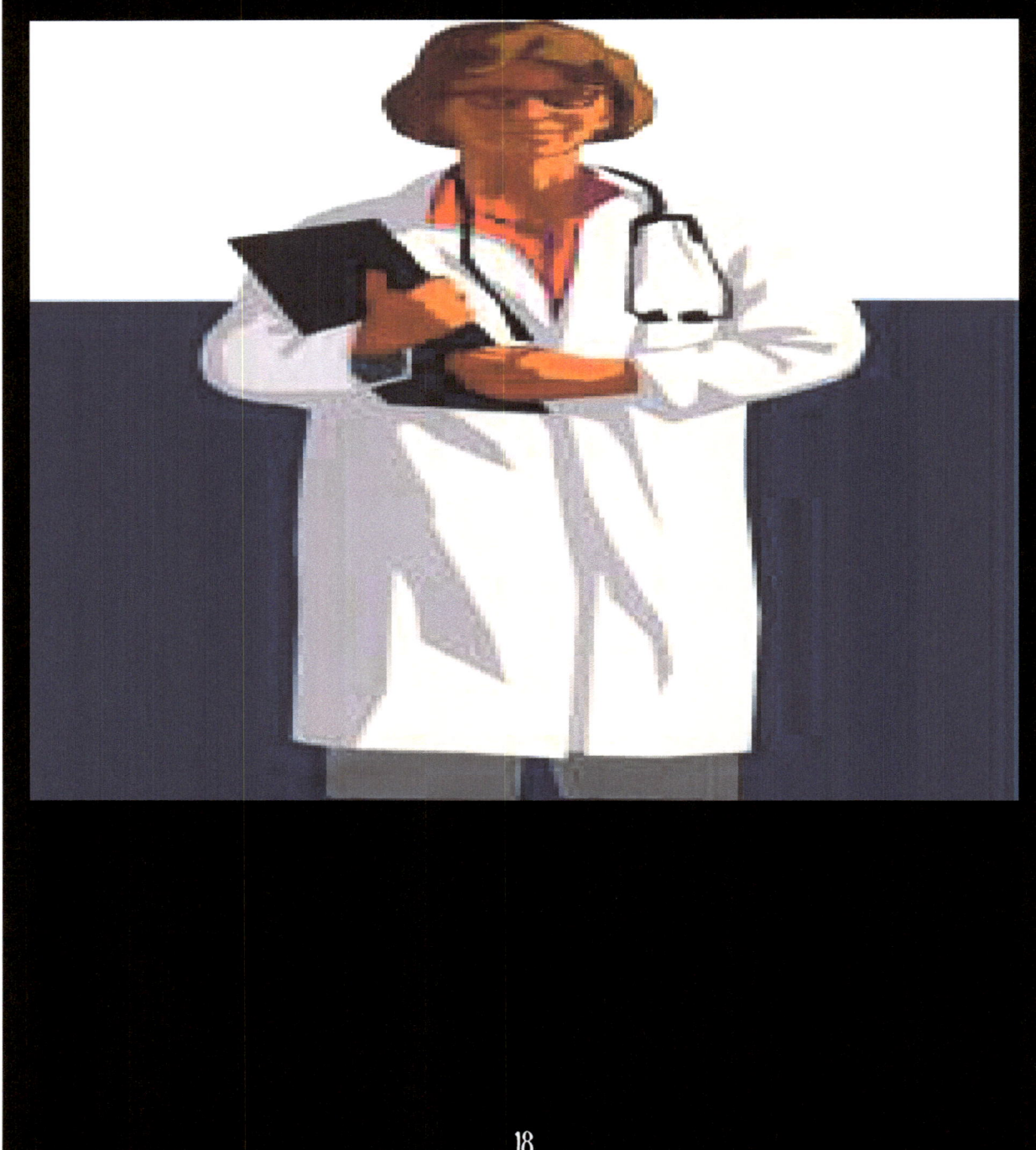

Fruits such as strawberries,water melons, grapes,Bananas, lemons,oranges, pears,apples and peaches, blueberries,blackberries,cantalopes and apples but you can only have small amounts as they too are natural in sugars. Lemons are best for diabetics though.

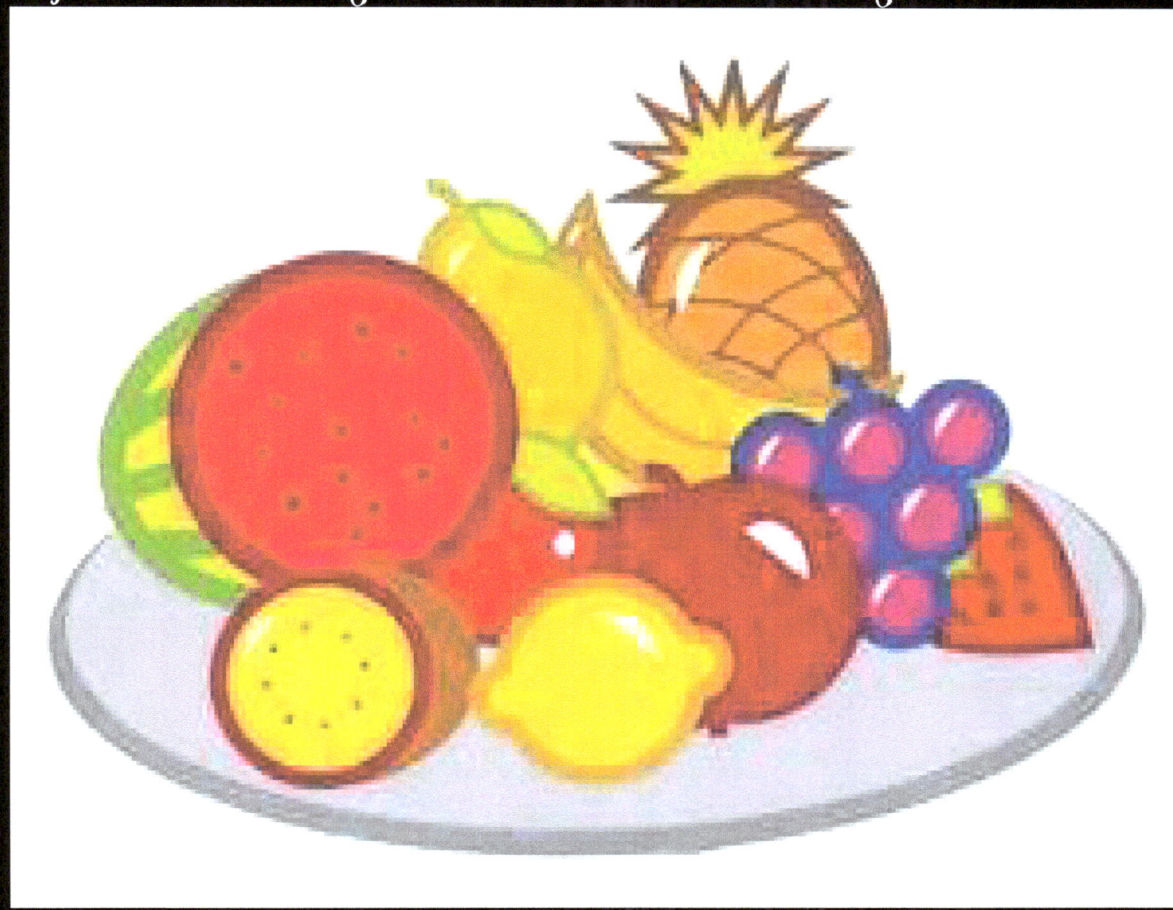

Getting the proper exercise is important to health and well balanced living. Some like jogging and running marathons. I do not recommend this though. As I like to say walk not run. Running can wear the body down and with it out goes your health. Jogging is not good for heels and feet either nor the heart. To make and say it best it is always better to go for morning and late afternoon walks a mile or two is all one needs.

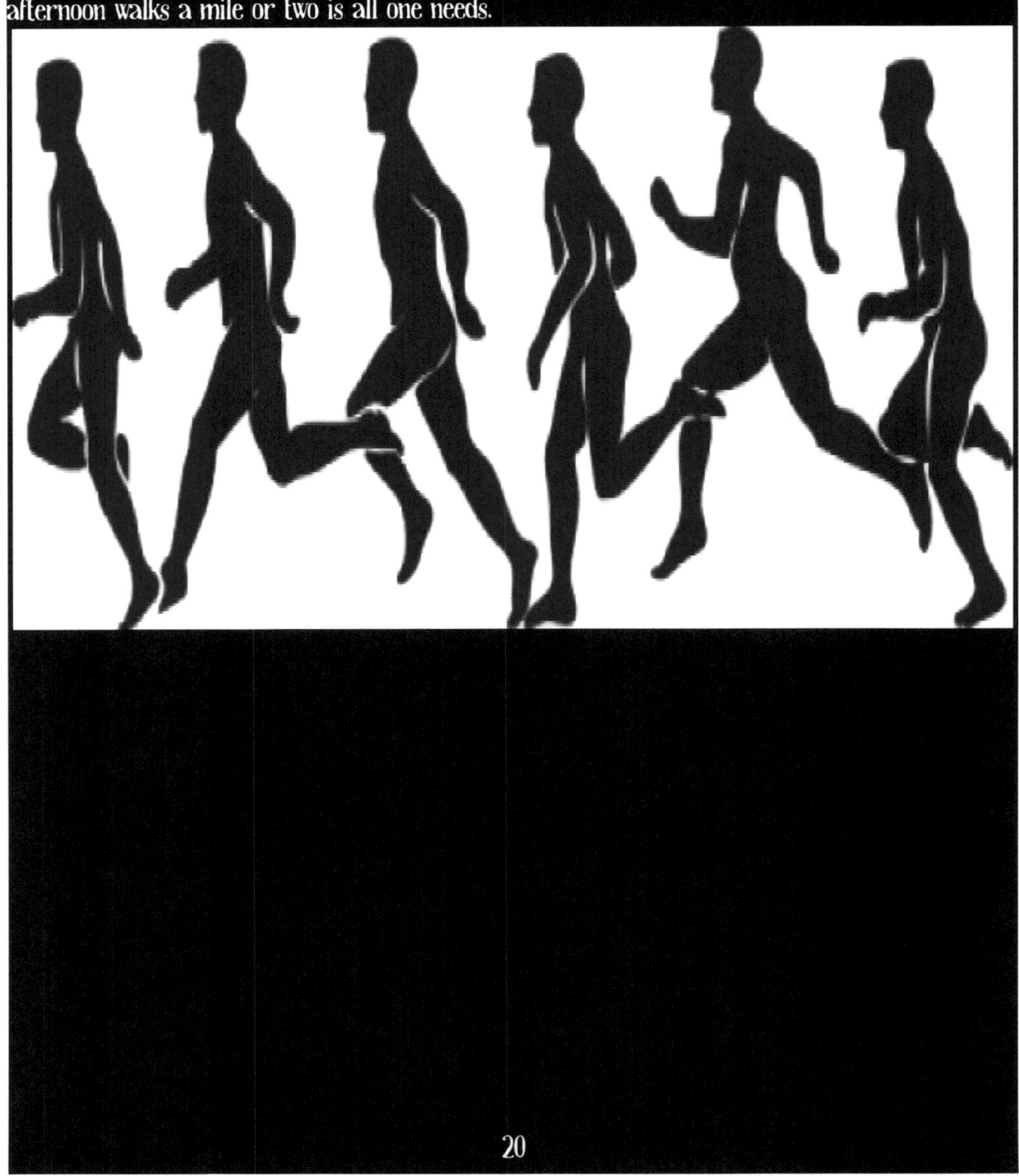

Now let us talk about choices for a moment. Choices is what you make of it. Simply I will say it, the will is yours to have and keep. What you say and do is from you. If you think positively and say over and over with to yourself I will win this battle to live against Diabetes then you will make it. But ultimately the choice is yours in the end...Choice live or die. Give up or beat it. You choose the road to go and follow. No one else can do it for you.

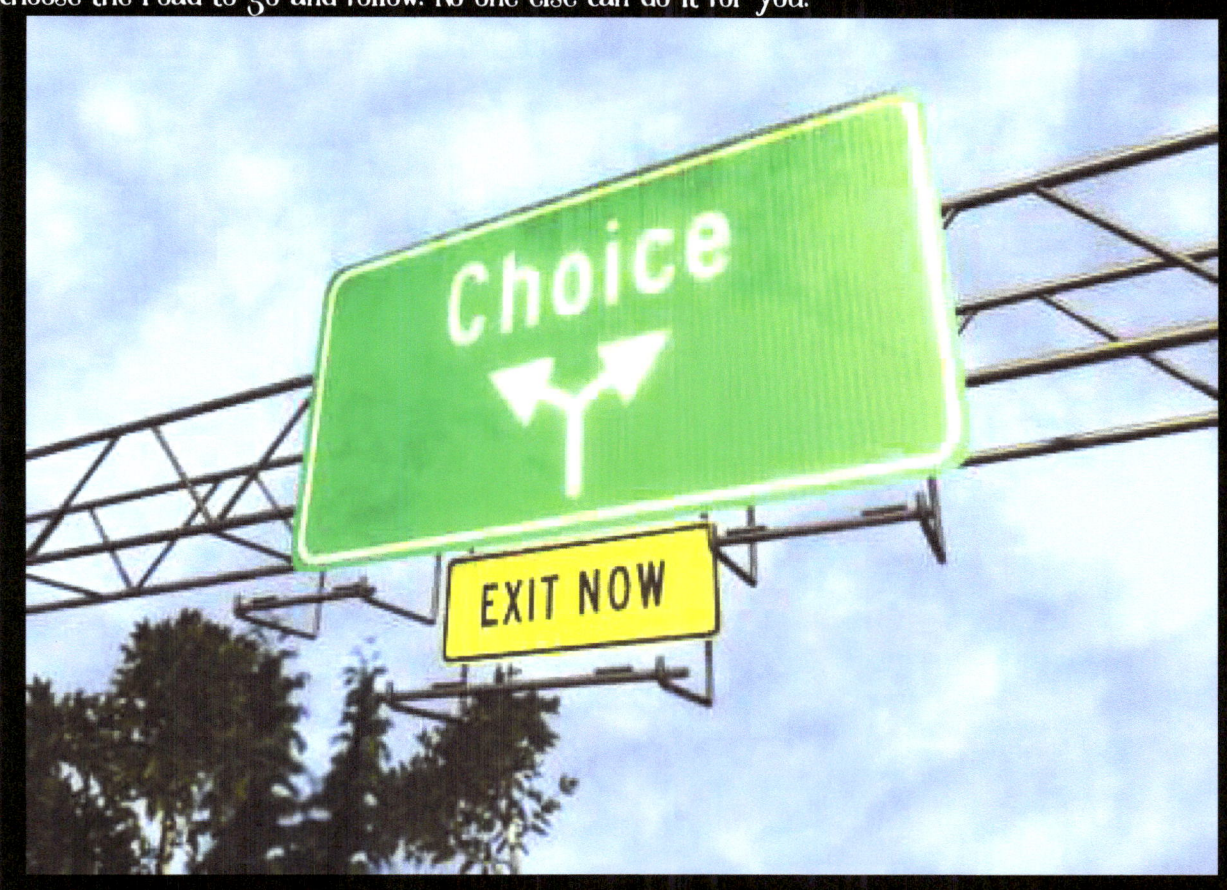

Having a good heart is all yours. Have a heart for those of us with diabetes because we're humans too and we want to live just like you do too. Look around you and you will see exactly what it is all about this world and being able to make it. Look around and go over to a stranger and shake hands with them and tell them you are glad to see them living. I'll bet you'll get more appreciation back from them than any so called friend or neighbors. A simple thank makes a person feel super in the day. It makes one feel good about themselves.

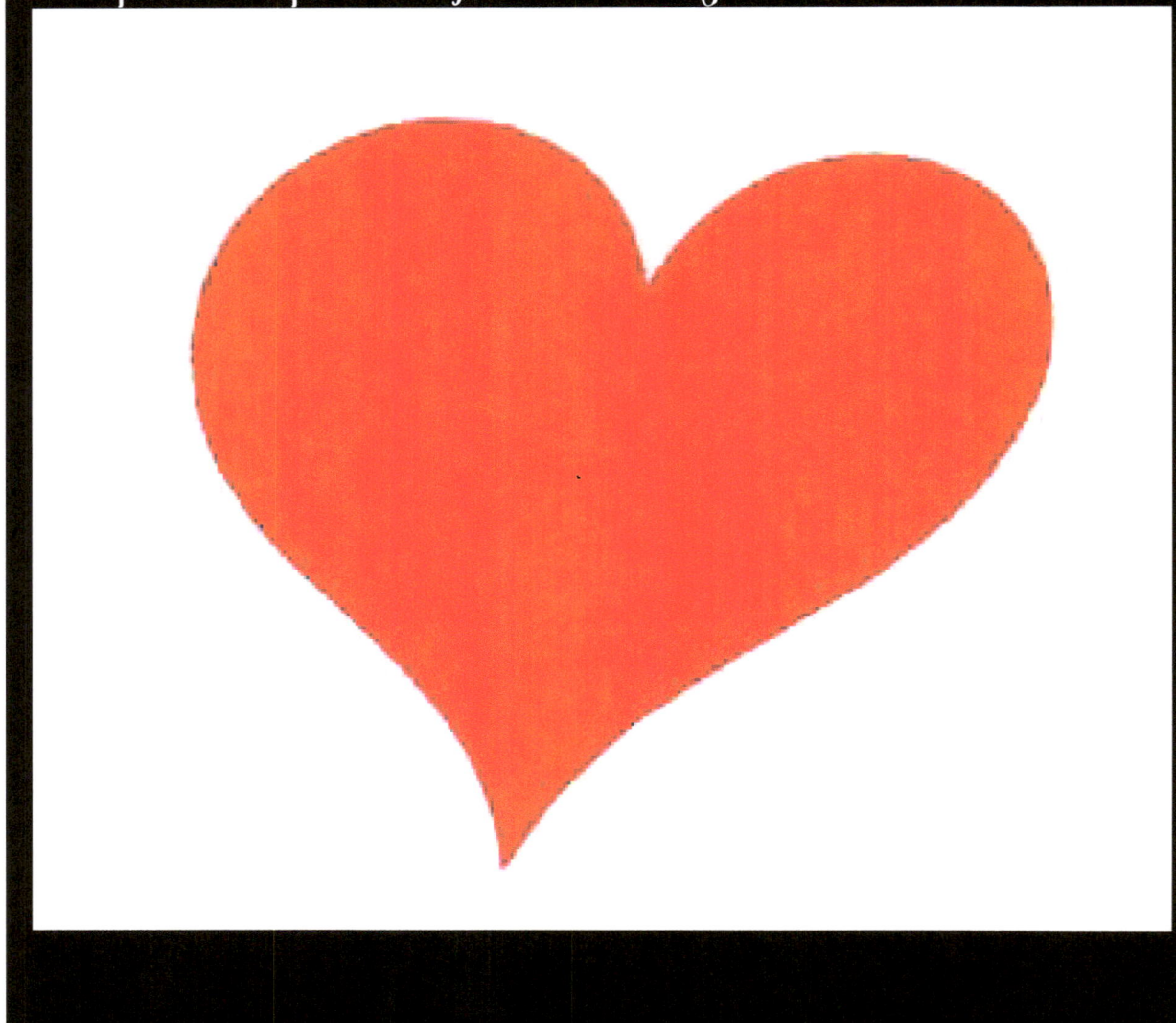

Remember testing your blood sugar levels on a day by day basis is one thing everyone needs to do. And keeping records is so important. One day those readings will become ever so needful to know and compare with when you go to the doctors. Above 120 will give you concerns and more so above 200 ldl.

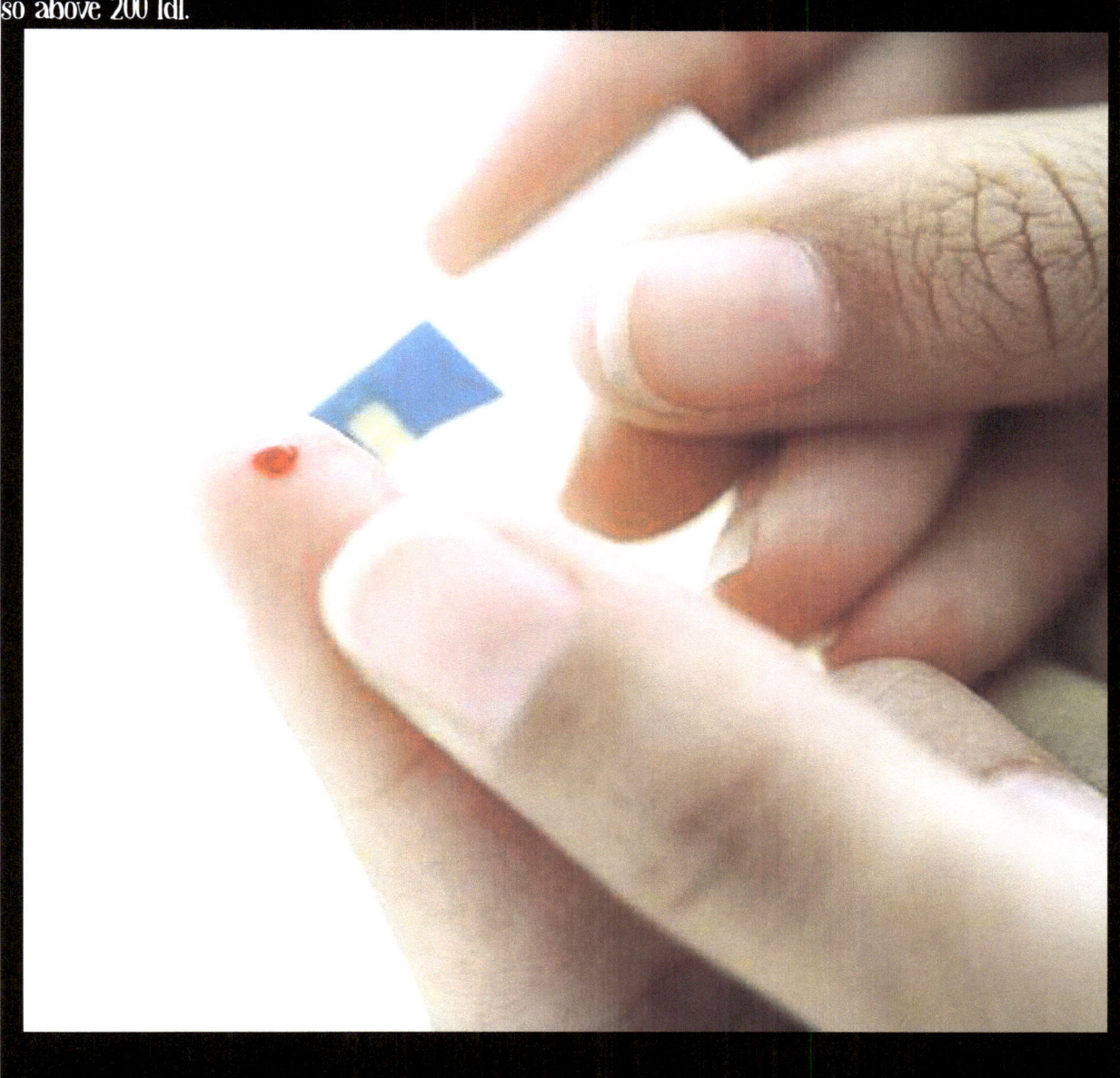

You need to ask yourself this is it mean more to have you in some coffin and family members or that loved one viewing your body and crying over you? Ask Am I going to win. Be confident about it and all you do and in the end you will find you are the winner. I'd rather be seen living and loved than be seen in that casket and being buried.

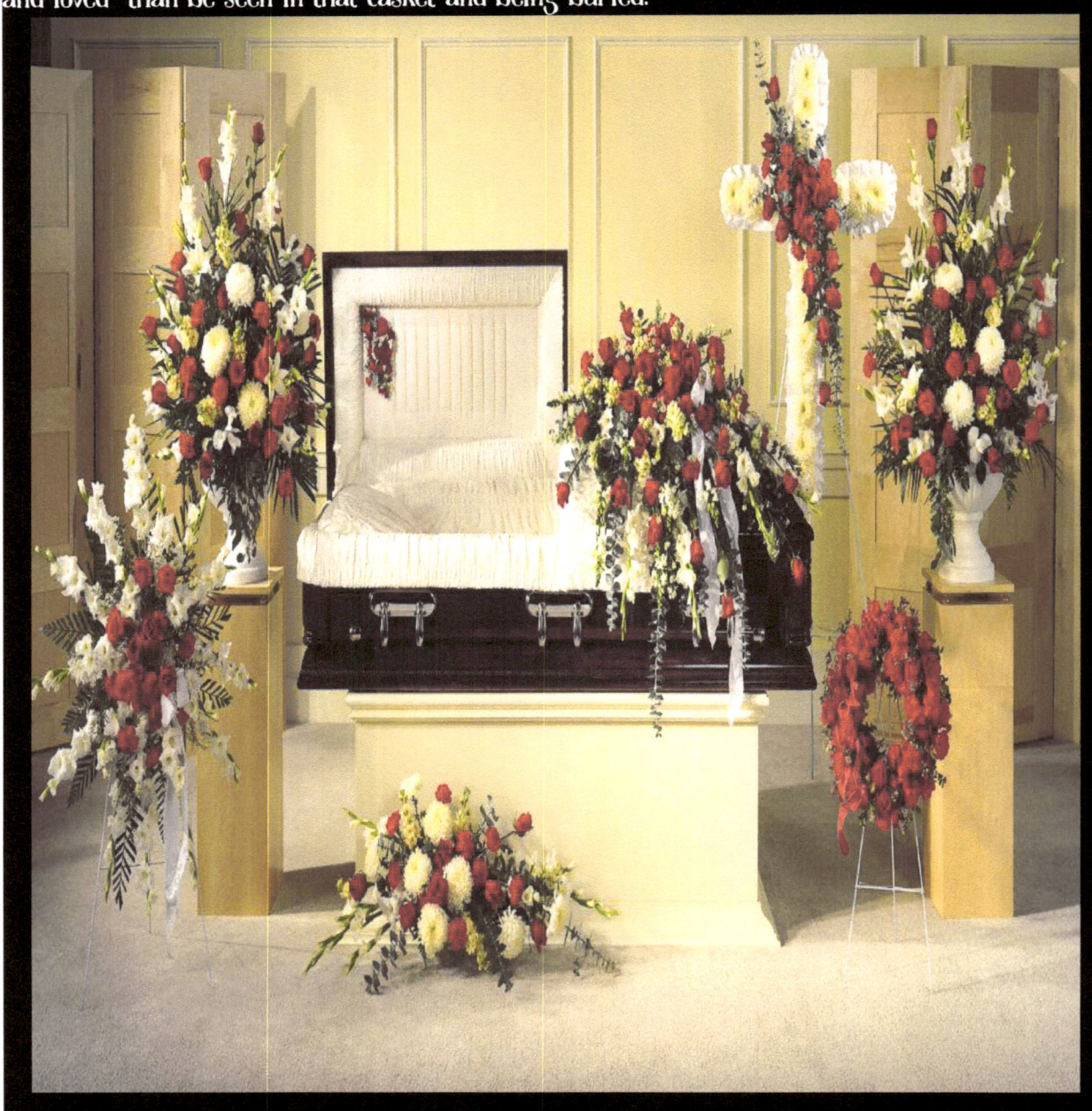

I know there are plenty of new medicines out there there today. And yet I am sure more will come. But I am speaking with courage and heart. There is a drug called TAk-875 and in studies it has shown promise and tremendous effects for lowering diabetes.It has been only down in clinical trials so far.   now that has stopped too. There needs to greater pressure on countries, our government and The FDA to make it easier to get this medication for diabetics. Not enough has been done for us diabetics. Laws have got to change for us. Grant it I would even be willing to be part of the studies.After all I have nothing to risk but tyr it. Lets put pressure on the FDA, government and pharmaceutical companies to make TAK-875 more accessible and easier t get for us diabetics. We need answers fast as to why this is not easy to receive.Do you agree with me diabetics.

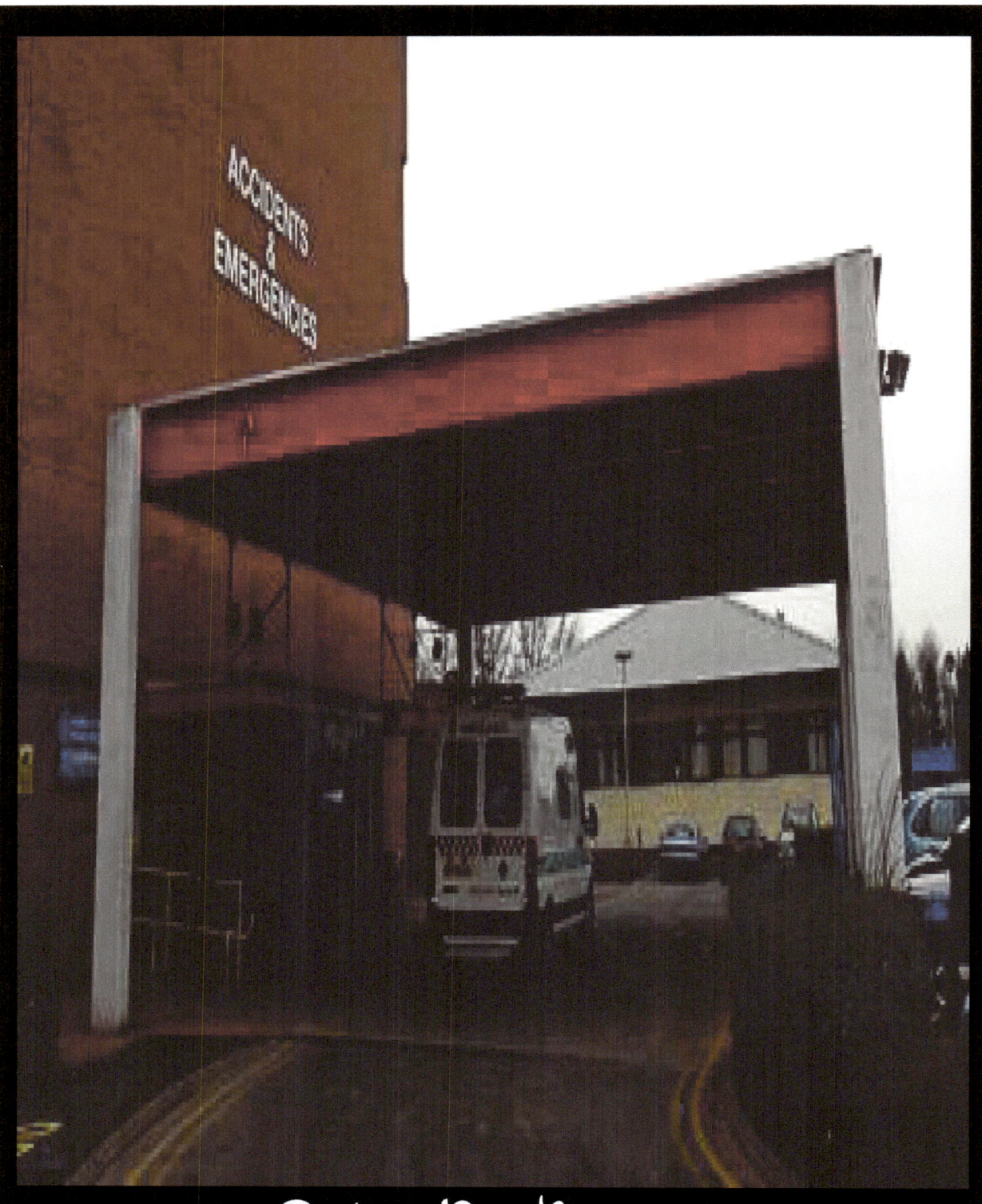

Diabetes Now Magazine

Written And Created By Cheyene Montana Lopez

www.ingramcontent.com/pod-product-compliance
Lightning Source LLC
Chambersburg PA
CBHW060820290526
45792CB00005BB/1729

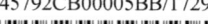